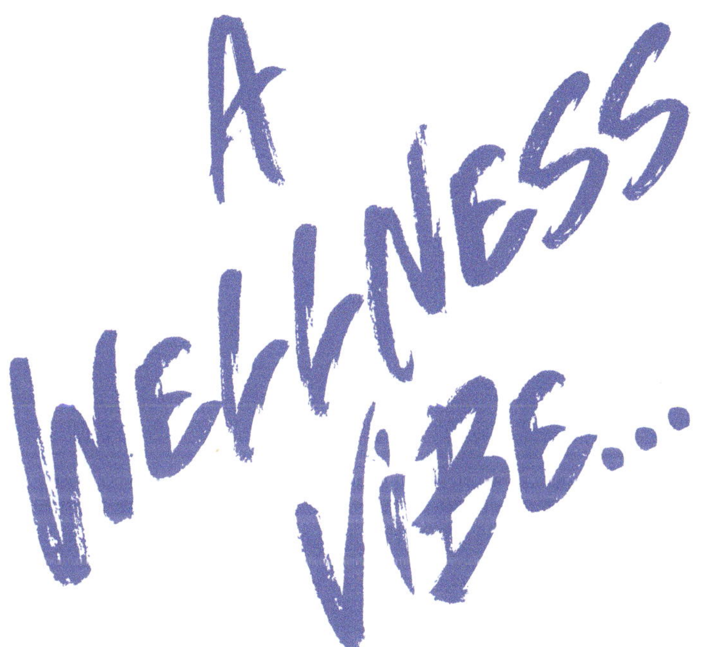

A WELLNESS VIBE...

created by
MELODIE NARAIN-BLACKWELL

For 30 days I will...

Month -

1	2	3	4	5
6	7	8	9	10
11	12	13	14	15
16	17	18	19	20
21	22	23	24	25
26	27	28	29	30

STARTED FROM:

______ / ______

NOW WE'RE HERE:

______ / ______

A WELLNESS VIBE...

wellness journal
created by
MELODIE NARAIN-BLACKWELL

Books may be purchased in bulk quantity by contacting the author.

Layout and Design created by
TBJ Brand Management Group

Published by Mynd Matters Publishing
715 Peachtree Street NE
Suites 100 & 200
Atlanta, GA 30308
www.myndmatterspublishing.com

978-1-957092-75-1 (pbk)

I NEED THESE TOOLS TO SUPPORT MY COMMITMENT.

TOP 3 THINGS THAT MIGHT HINDER MY PROGRESS ARE?

MY SUPPORT TEAM:

I WILL COMPLETE MY 30 DAY COMMITMENT BECAUSE...

My Healthy Habits are...

EAT BREAKFAST

SELF-CARE

EXERCISE DAILY

DRINKING WATER

MENTAL HEALTH BREAK

POSITIVE THOUGHTS

MEAL PLANNING

GOING OFF THE GRID

REST MORE

SAVE MORE

LAUGH OUT LOUD

TREAT YOURSELF

TAKE TIME FOR YOURSELF

Creating healthy habits for a healthier you!

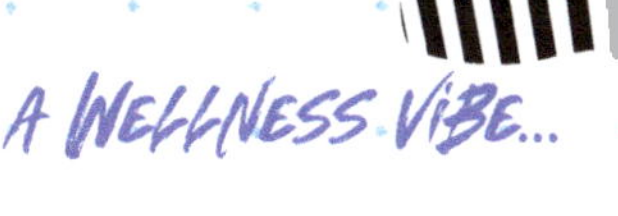

FEEL GOOD FOODS... (Best foods for my overall health that don't negative responses.)

FEEL BAD FOODS... (Foods that trigger symptoms that have negative responses.)

GOOD MOOD FOODS... (Snacks that keep me FUNctional.)

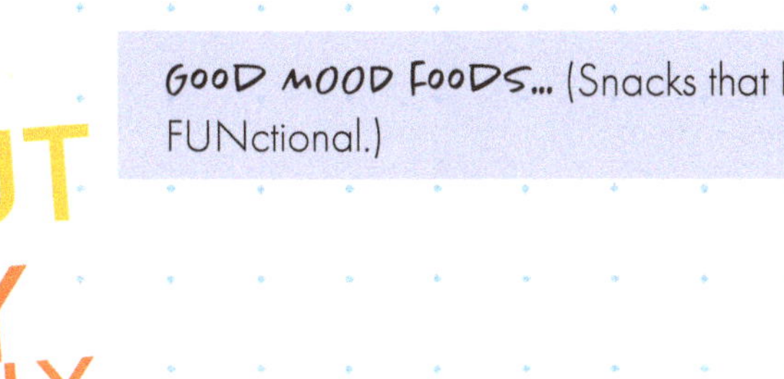

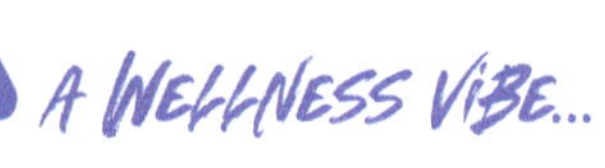

Health is wealth… let's get rich!

WELLNESS REMINDER:

HOW MUCH WATER DID YOU DRINK TODAY?

Health experts commonly recommend eight 8-ounce glasses, which equals about 2 liters, or half a gallon a day.

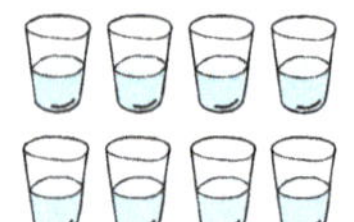

MENTAL CHECK-IN:

HOW ARE WE FEELING TODAY?

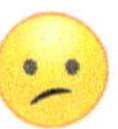

TOP PRIORITIES TODAY:

- ☐
- ☐
- ☐
- ☐
- ☐

CONNECT WITH:

- ☐
- ☐
- ☐
- ☐
- ☐

HOT
LIST

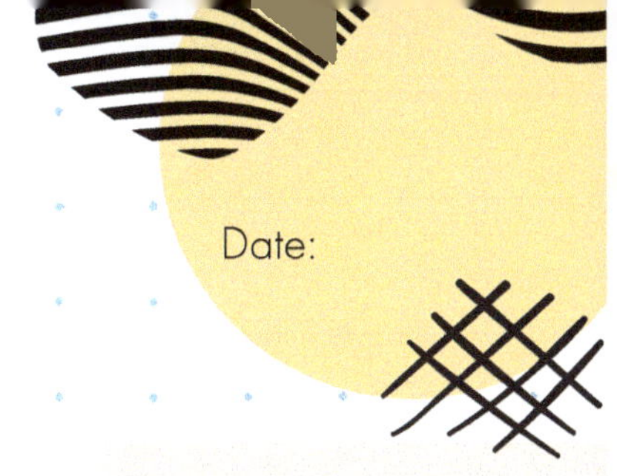

Date:

REMINDERS:

TARGET LIST FOR TOMORROW:

A Wellness Vibe...

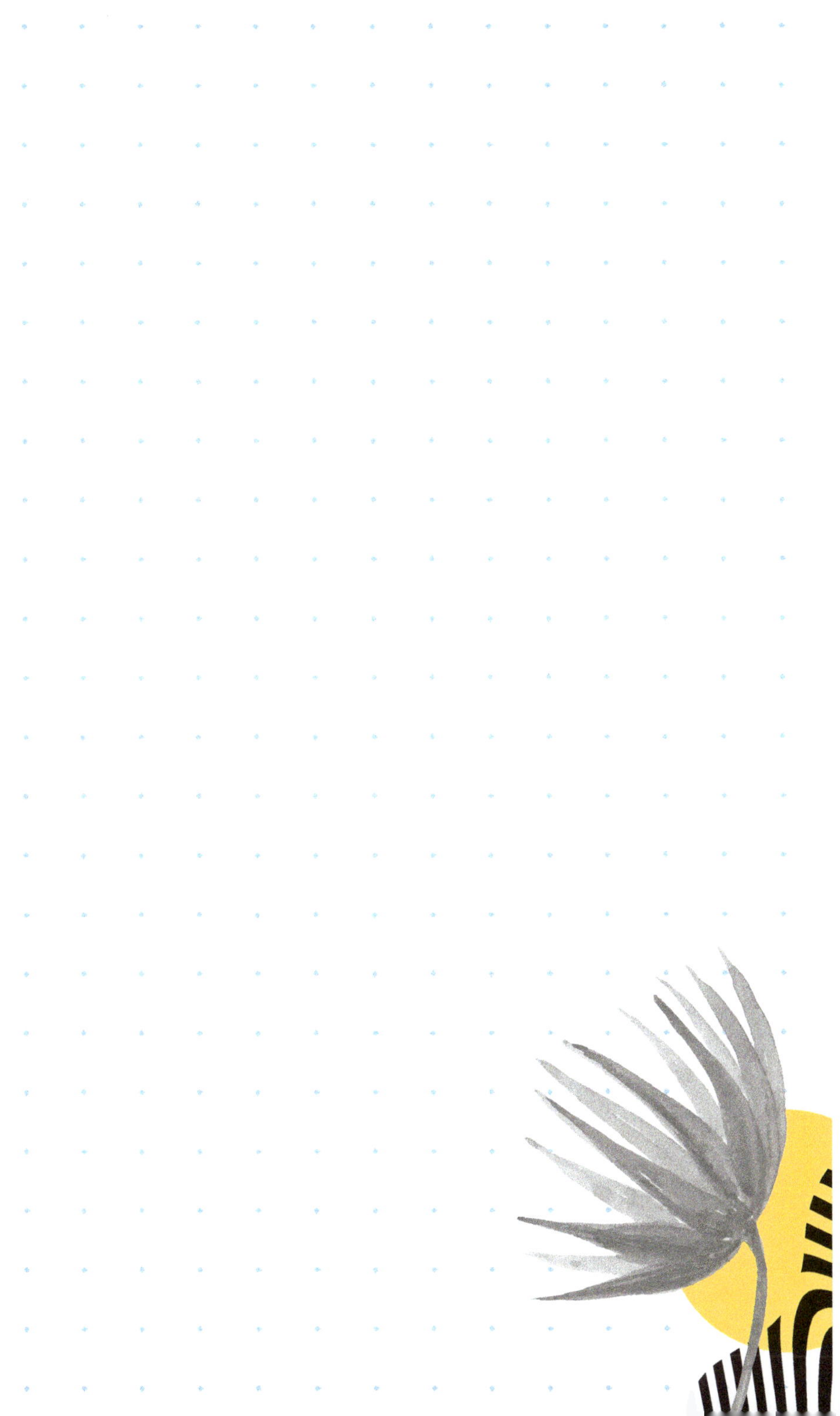

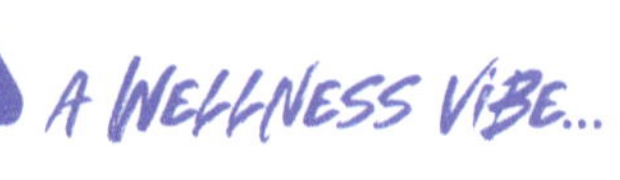

DAILY ROUTINE.

Health is wealth... let's get rich!

WELLNESS REMINDER:

HOW MUCH WATER DID YOU DRINK TODAY?

Health experts commonly recommend eight 8-ounce glasses, which equals about 2 liters, or half a gallon a day.

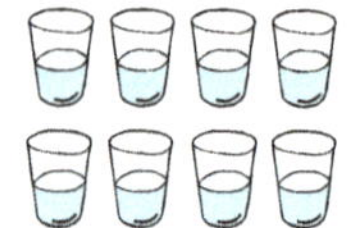

MENTAL CHECK-IN:

HOW ARE WE FEELING TODAY?

TOP PRIORITIES TODAY:

CONNECT WITH:

HOT
LIST

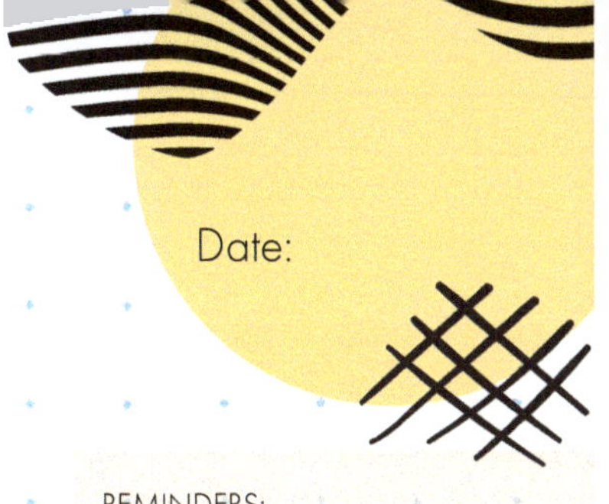

Date:

REMINDERS:

TARGET LIST FOR TOMORROW:

A Wellness Vibe...

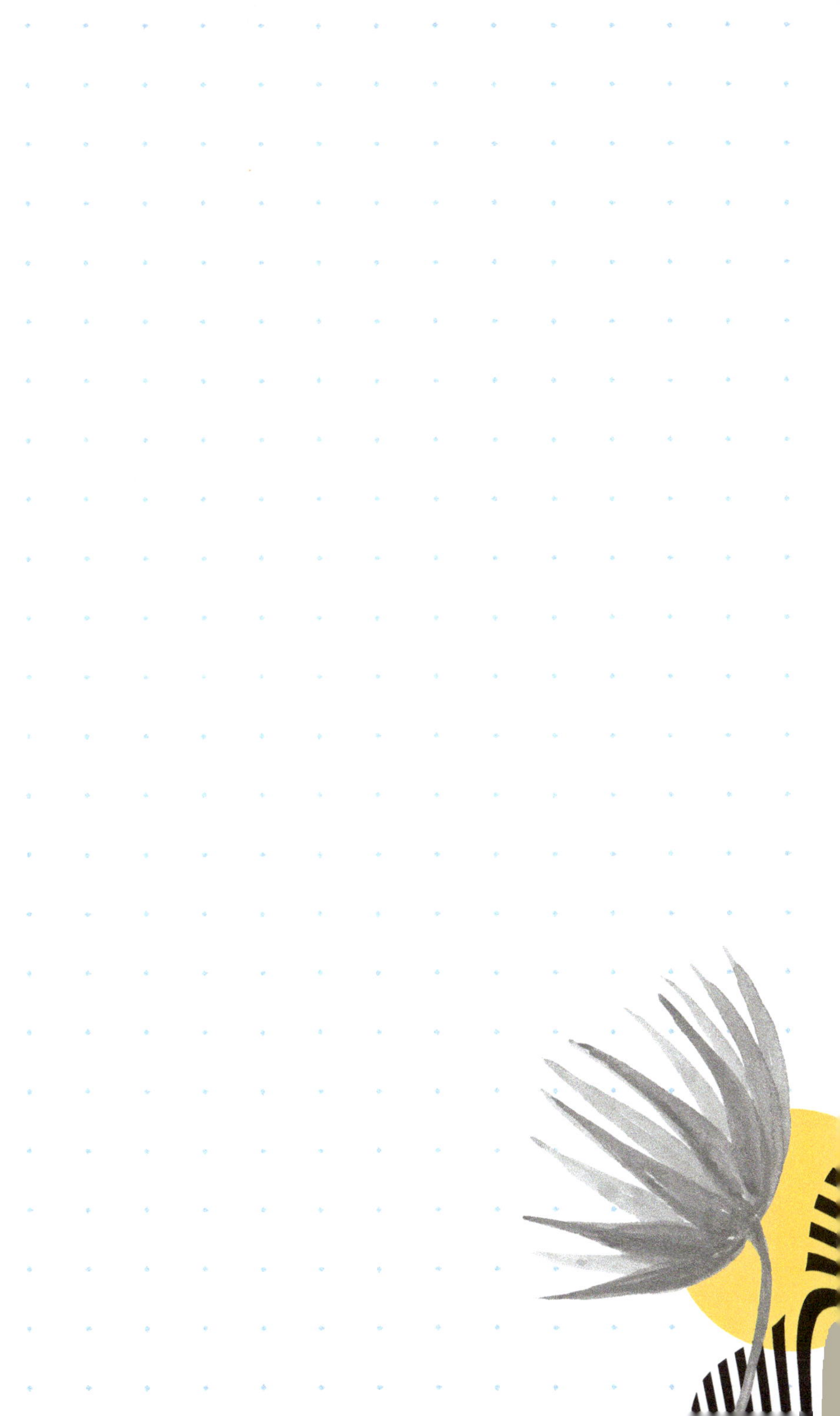

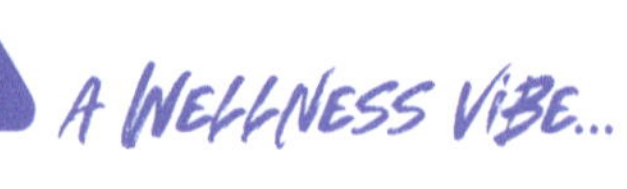

DAILY ROUTINE.

Health is wealth... let's get rich!

WELLNESS REMINDER:

HOW MUCH WATER DID YOU DRINK TODAY?

Health experts commonly recommend eight 8-ounce glasses, which equals about 2 liters, or half a gallon a day.

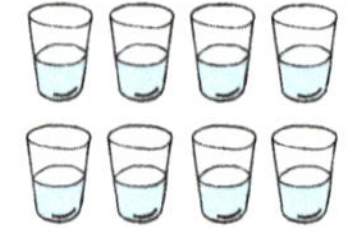

MENTAL CHECK-IN:

HOW ARE WE FEELING TODAY?

TOP PRIORITIES TODAY:

- ☐
- ☐
- ☐
- ☐
- ☐

CONNECT WITH:

- ☐
- ☐
- ☐
- ☐
- ☐

HOT LIST

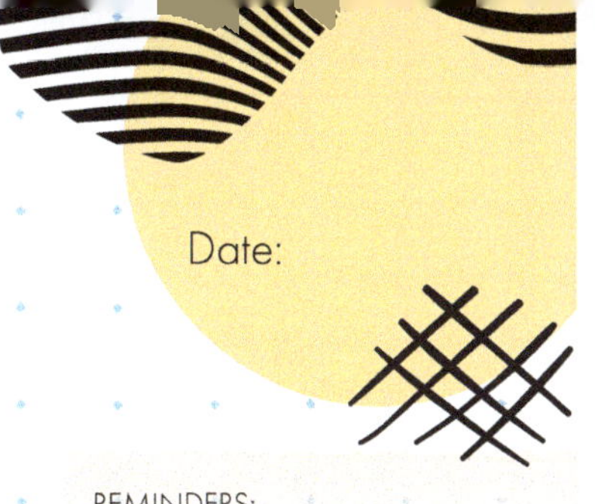

Date:

REMINDERS:

TARGET LIST FOR TOMORROW:

NOTES

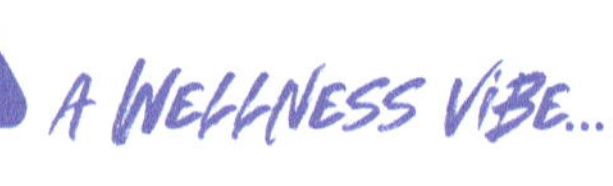

Health is wealth... let's get rich!

WELLNESS REMINDER:

HOW MUCH WATER DID YOU DRINK TODAY?

Health experts commonly recommend eight 8-ounce glasses, which equals about 2 liters, or half a gallon a day.

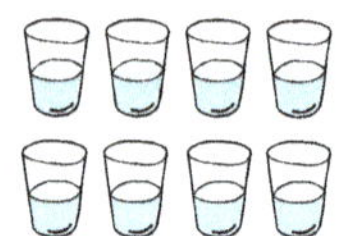

MENTAL CHECK-IN:

HOW ARE WE FEELING TODAY?

TOP PRIORITIES TODAY:

- ☐
- ☐
- ☐
- ☐
- ☐

CONNECT WITH:

- ☐
- ☐
- ☐
- ☐
- ☐

HOT LIST

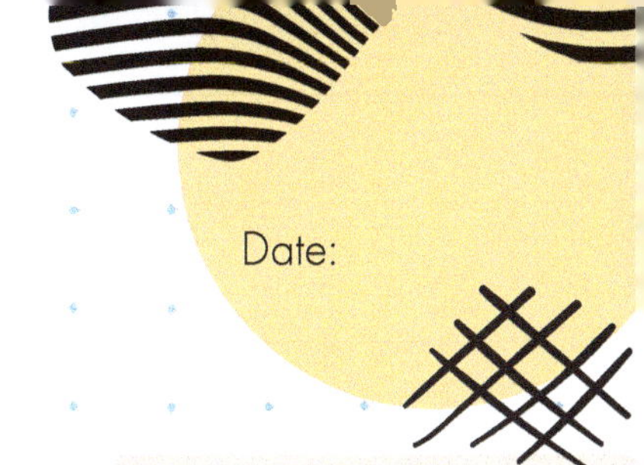

Date:

REMINDERS:

TARGET LIST FOR TOMORROW:

A Wellness Vibe...

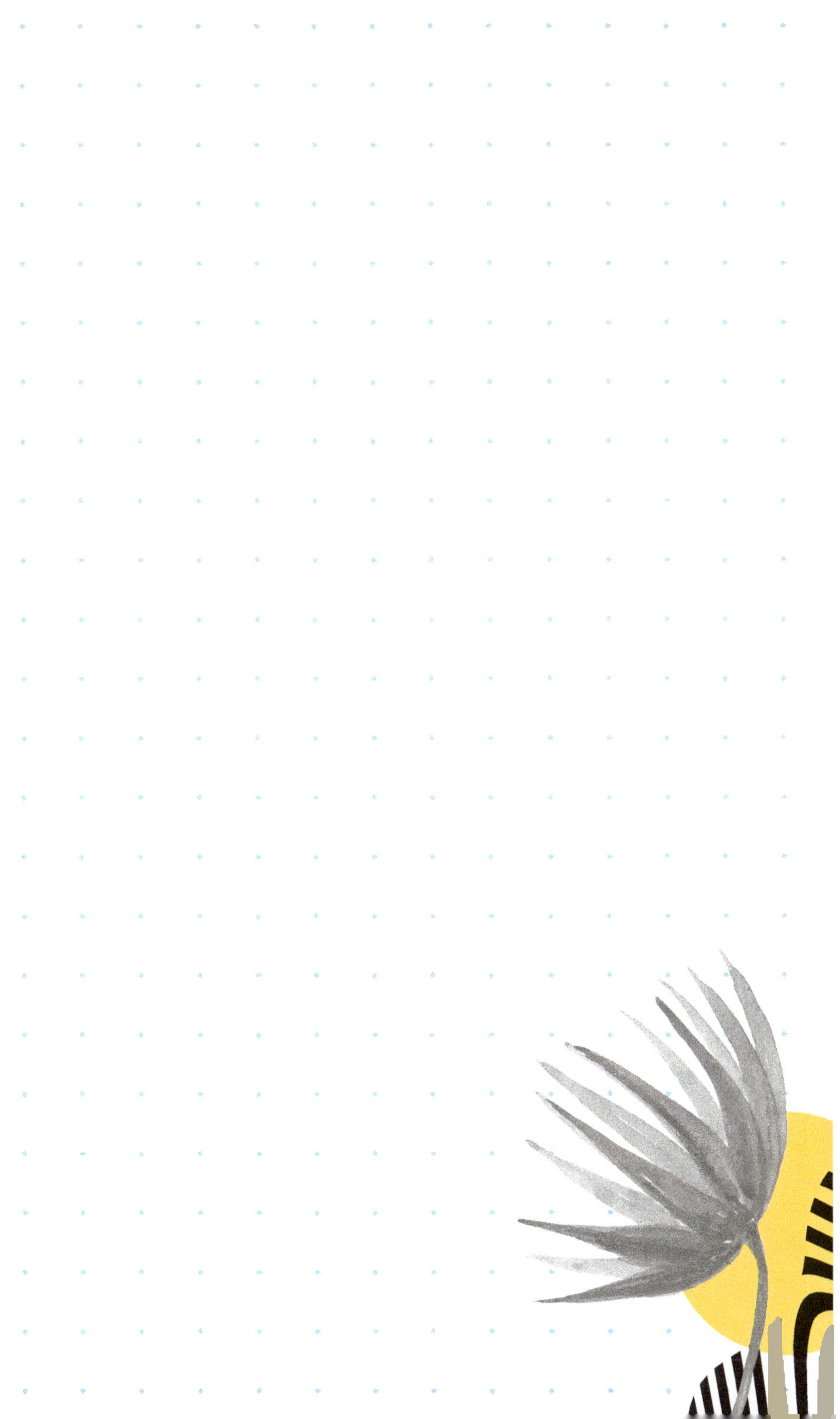

A WELLNESS VIBE...

DAILY ROUTINE.

Health is wealth... let's get rich!

WELLNESS REMINDER:

HOW MUCH WATER DID YOU DRINK TODAY?

Health experts commonly recommend eight 8-ounce glasses, which equals about 2 liters, or half a gallon a day.

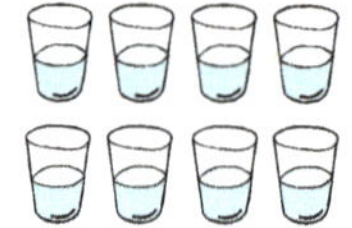

MENTAL CHECK-IN:

HOW ARE WE FEELING TODAY?

TOP PRIORITIES TODAY:

- ☐
- ☐
- ☐
- ☐
- ☐

CONNECT WITH:

- ☐
- ☐
- ☐
- ☐
- ☐

HOT LIST

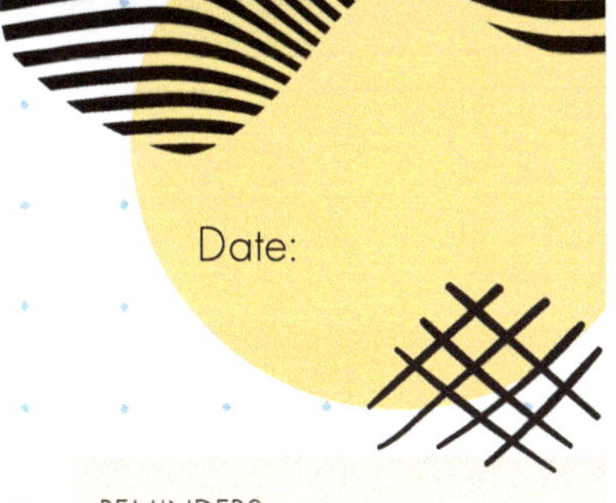

Date:

REMINDERS:

TARGET LIST FOR TOMORROW:

A Wellness Vibe...

NOTES

A WELLNESS VIBE...

DAILY ROUTINE.

Health is wealth... let's get rich!

WELLNESS REMINDER:

HOW MUCH WATER DID YOU DRINK TODAY?

Health experts commonly recommend eight 8-ounce glasses, which equals about 2 liters, or half a gallon a day.

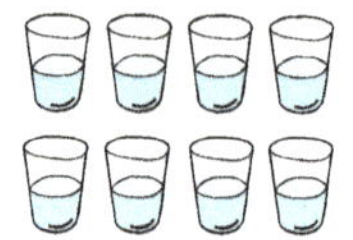

MENTAL CHECK-IN:

HOW ARE WE FEELING TODAY?

TOP PRIORITIES TODAY:

- ☐
- ☐
- ☐
- ☐
- ☐

CONNECT WITH:

- ☐
- ☐
- ☐
- ☐
- ☐

HOT LIST

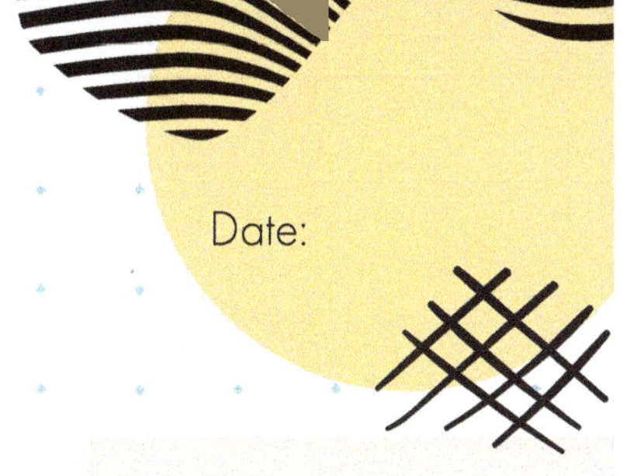

Date:

REMINDERS:

TARGET LIST FOR TOMORROW:

NOTES

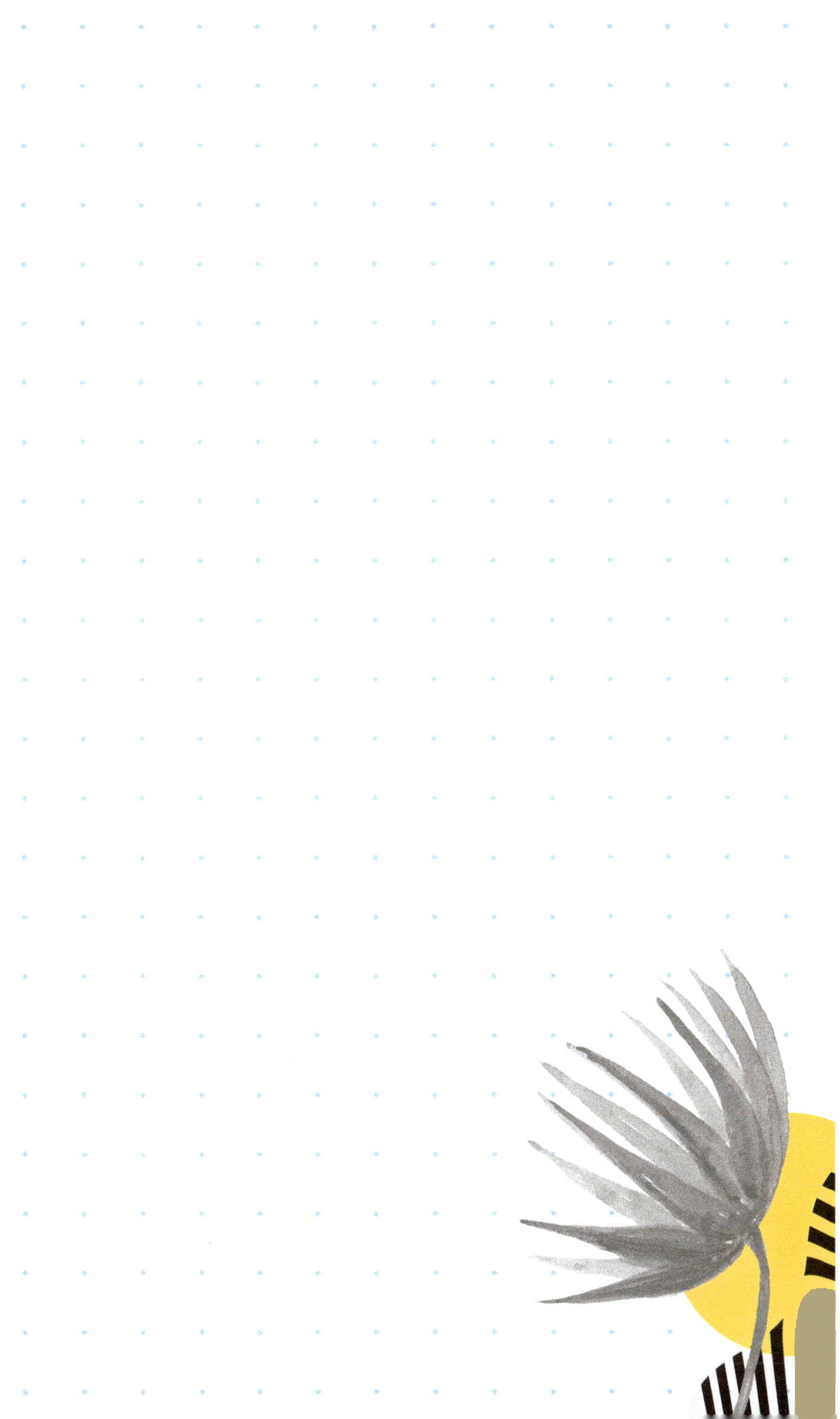

DAILY ROUTINE.

Health is wealth... let's get rich!

WELLNESS REMINDER:

HOW MUCH WATER DID YOU DRINK TODAY?

Health experts commonly recommend eight 8-ounce glasses, which equals about 2 liters, or half a gallon a day.

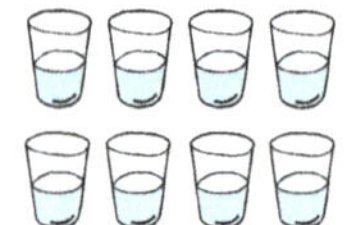

MENTAL CHECK-IN:

HOW ARE WE FEELING TODAY?

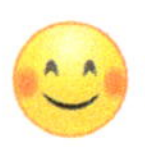

TOP PRIORITIES TODAY:

- [ ]
- [ ]
- [ ]
- [ ]
- [ ]

CONNECT WITH:

- [ ]
- [ ]
- [ ]
- [ ]
- [ ]

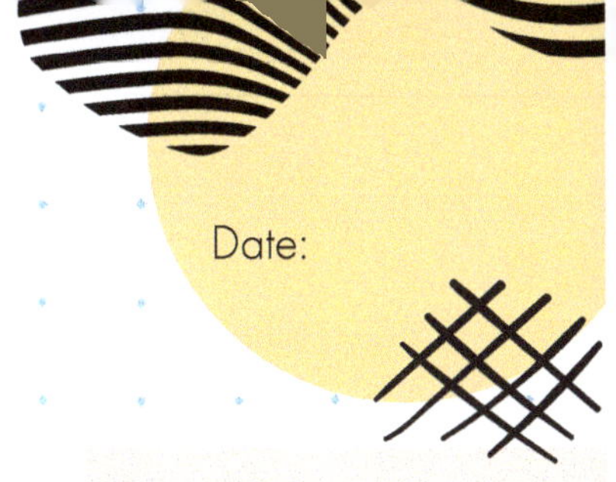

Date:

REMINDERS:

TARGET LIST FOR TOMORROW:

NOTES

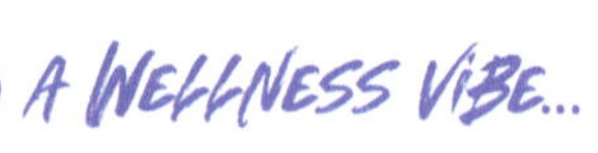

DAILY ROUTINE.

Health is wealth... let's get rich!

WELLNESS REMINDER:

HOW MUCH WATER DID YOU DRINK TODAY?

Health experts commonly recommend eight 8-ounce glasses, which equals about 2 liters, or half a gallon a day.

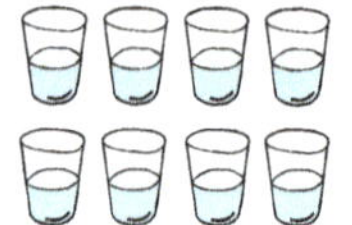

MENTAL CHECK-IN:

HOW ARE WE FEELING TODAY?

TOP PRIORITIES TODAY:

- [ ]
- [ ]
- [ ]
- [ ]
- [ ]

CONNECT WITH:

- [ ]
- [ ]
- [ ]
- [ ]
- [ ]

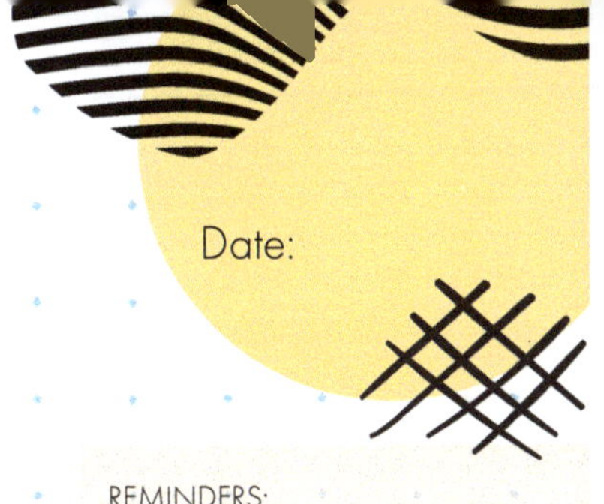

Date:

REMINDERS:

TARGET LIST FOR TOMORROW:

A Wellness Vibe...

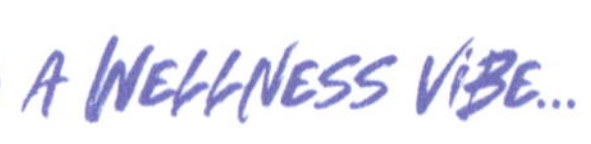 A WELLNESS VIBE...

Health is wealth... let's get rich!

WELLNESS REMINDER:

HOW MUCH WATER DID YOU DRINK TODAY?

Health experts commonly recommend eight 8-ounce glasses, which equals about 2 liters, or half a gallon a day.

MENTAL CHECK-IN:

HOW ARE WE FEELING TODAY?

TOP PRIORITIES TODAY:

CONNECT WITH:

HOT LIST

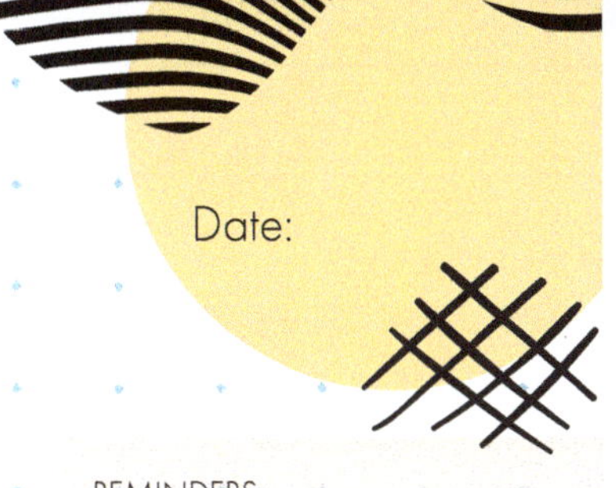

Date:

REMINDERS:

TARGET LIST FOR TOMORROW:

NOTES

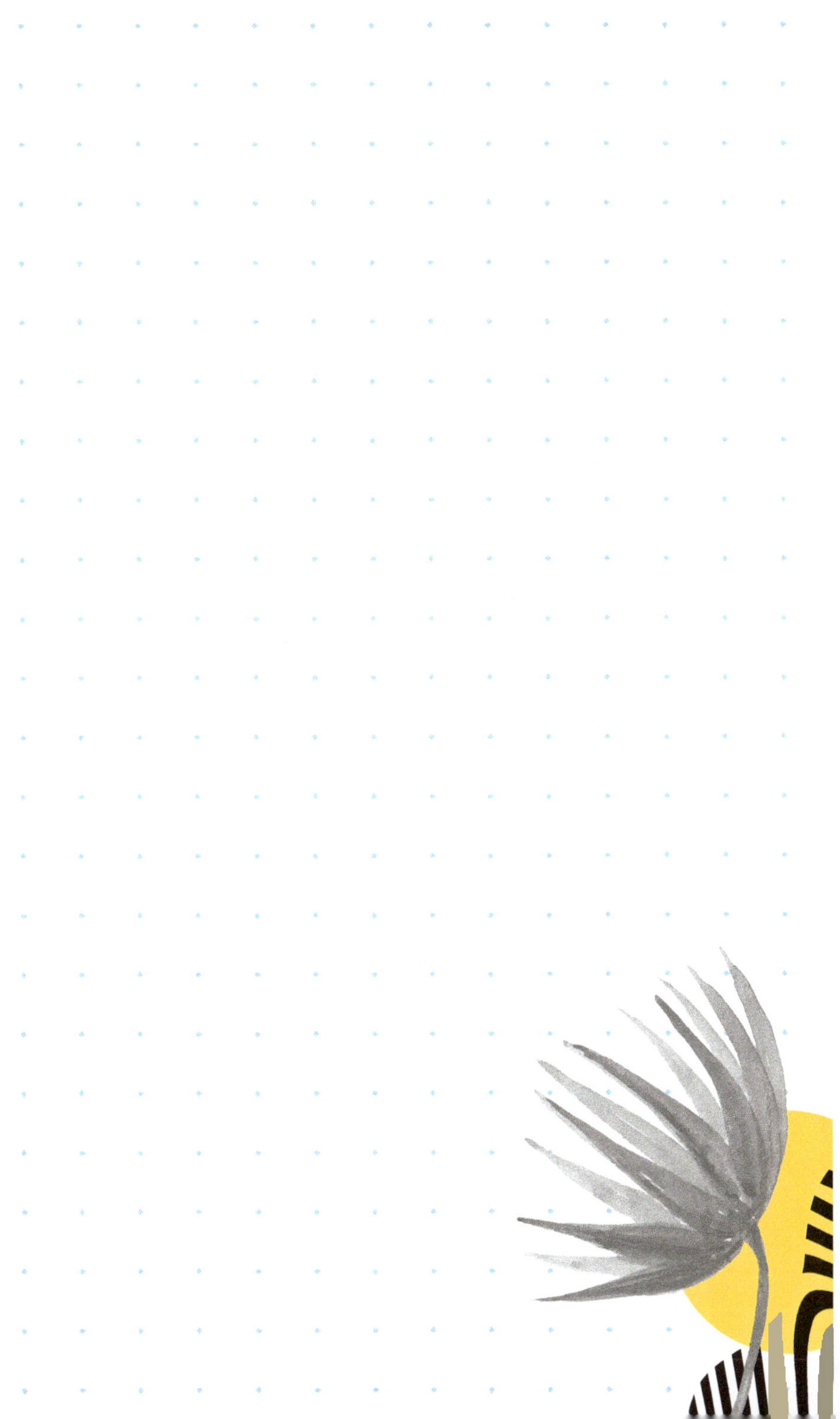

DAILY ROUTINE.

Health is wealth... let's get rich!

WELLNESS REMINDER:

HOW MUCH WATER DID YOU DRINK TODAY?

Health experts commonly recommend eight 8-ounce glasses, which equals about 2 liters, or half a gallon a day.

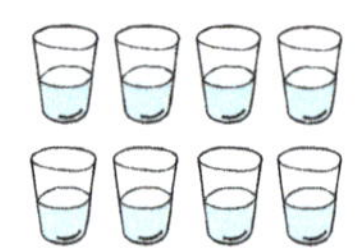

MENTAL CHECK-IN:

HOW ARE WE FEELING TODAY?

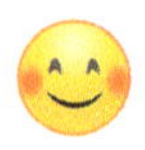

TOP PRIORITIES TODAY:

- ☐
- ☐
- ☐
- ☐
- ☐

CONNECT WITH:

- ☐
- ☐
- ☐
- ☐
- ☐

HOT
LIST

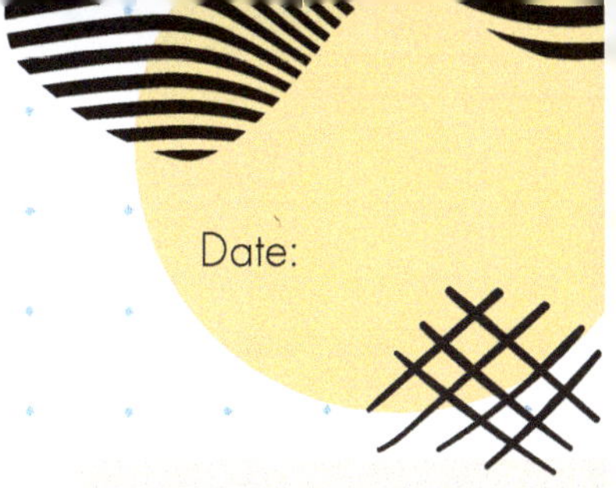

Date:

REMINDERS:

TARGET LIST FOR TOMORROW:

A Wellness Vibe...

A Wellness Vibe...

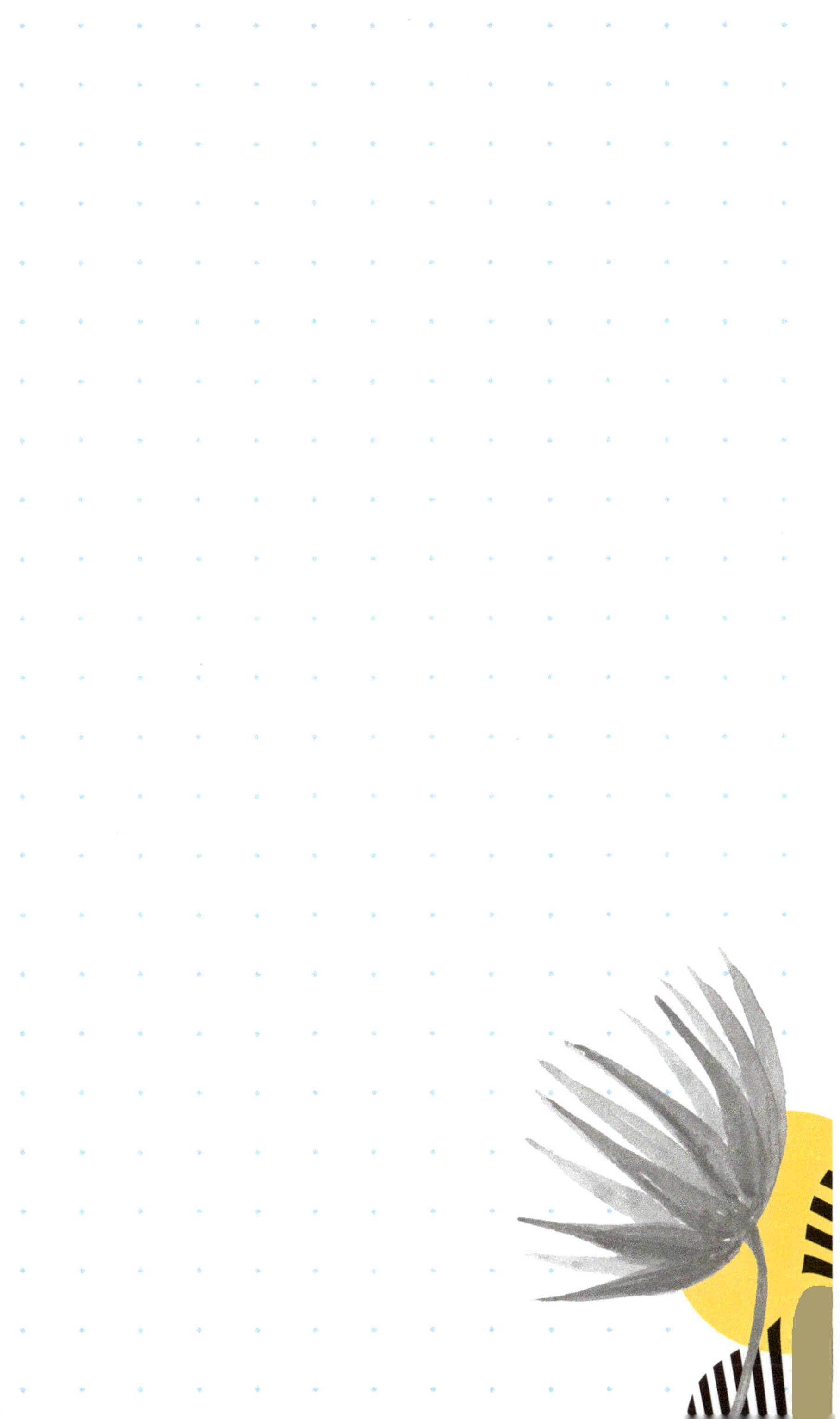

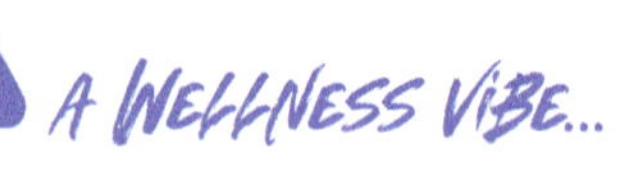

DAILY ROUTINE.

Health is wealth... let's get rich!

WELLNESS REMINDER:

HOW MUCH WATER DID YOU DRINK TODAY?

Health experts commonly recommend eight 8-ounce glasses, which equals about 2 liters, or half a gallon a day.

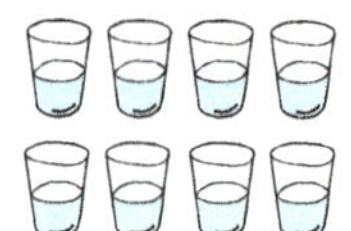

MENTAL CHECK-IN:

HOW ARE WE FEELING TODAY?

TOP PRIORITIES TODAY:

- ☐
- ☐
- ☐
- ☐
- ☐

CONNECT WITH:

- ☐
- ☐
- ☐
- ☐
- ☐

HOT LIST

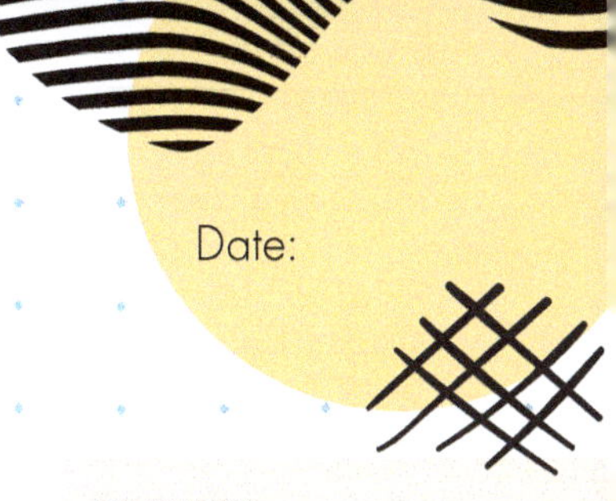

Date:

REMINDERS:

TARGET LIST FOR TOMORROW:

A WELLNESS VIBE...

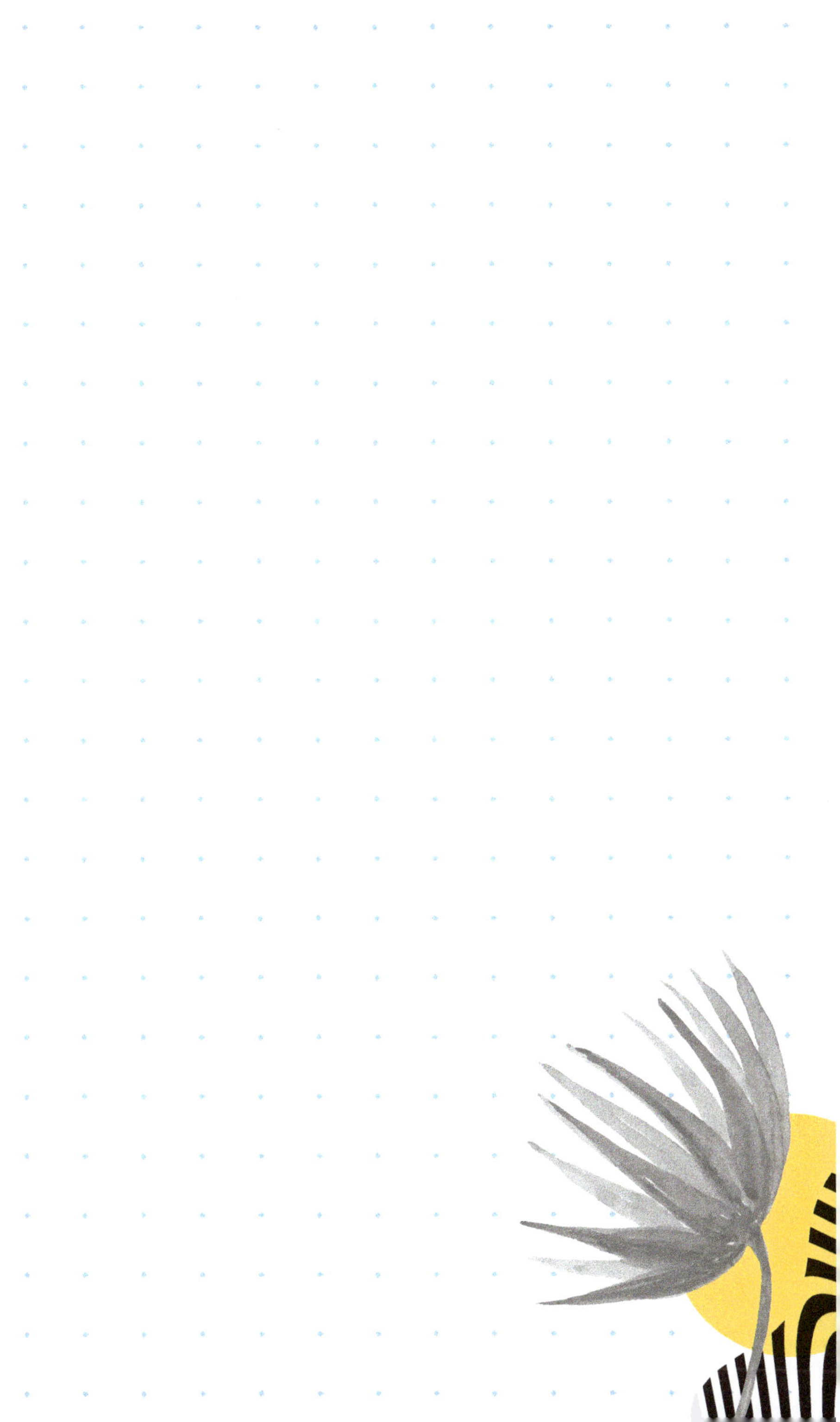

A WELLNESS VIBE...

NOTES

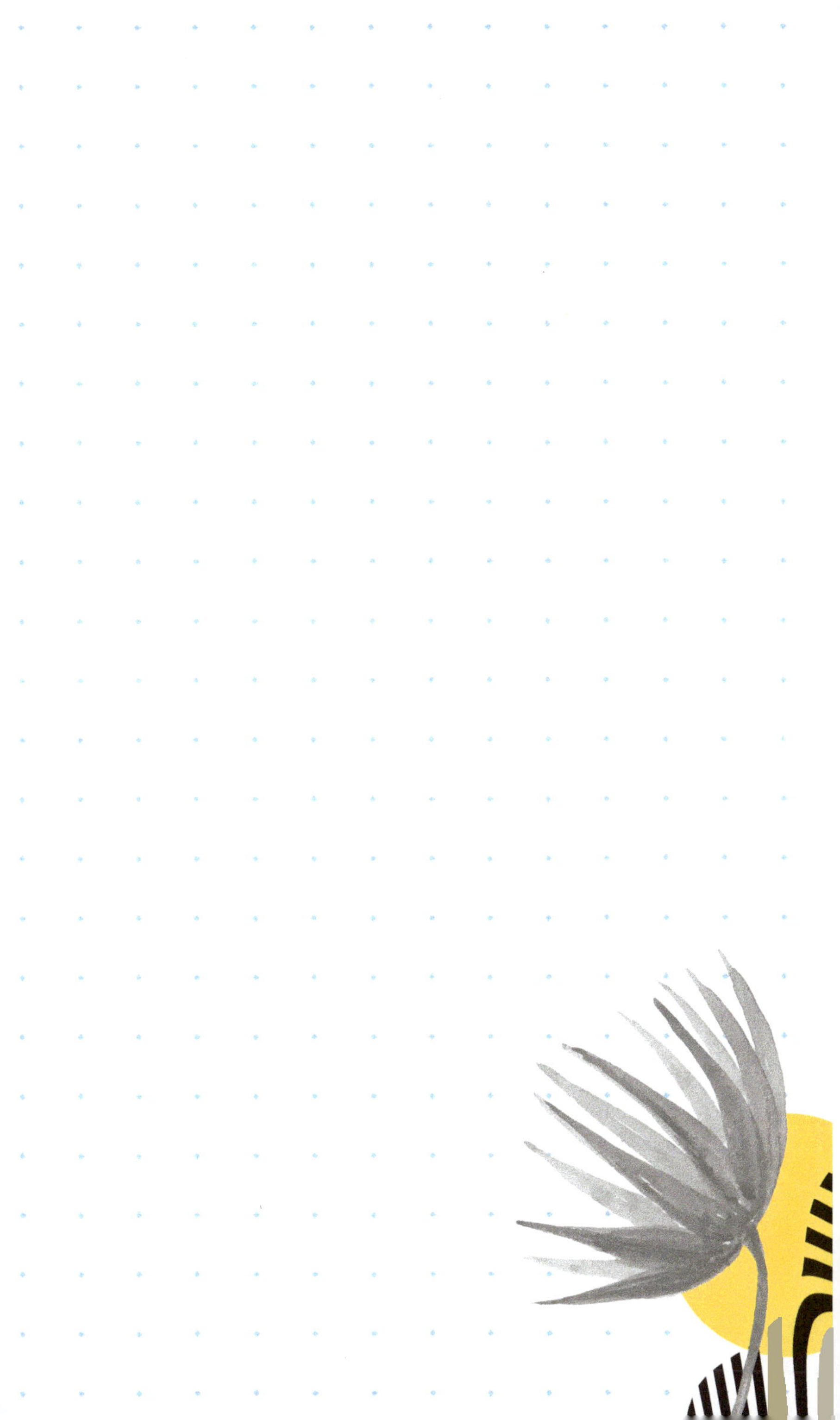

A Wellness Vibe...

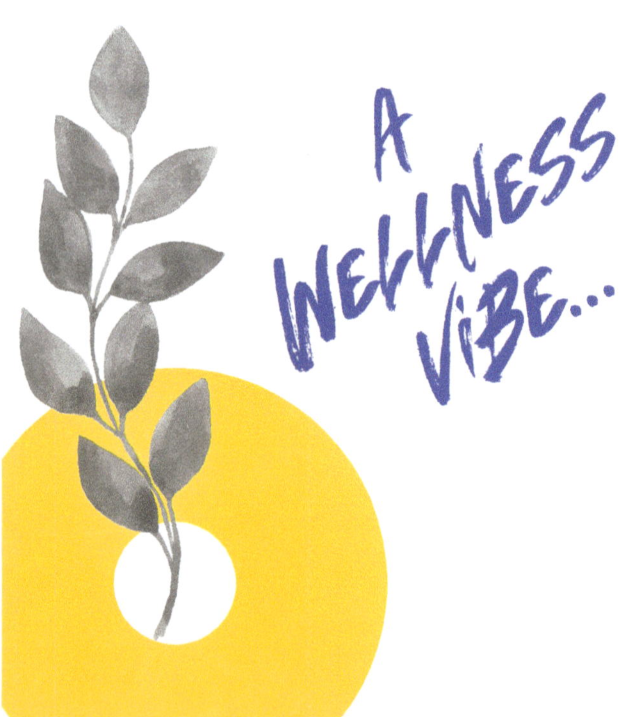
A
WELLNESS
VIBE...